Bone Broth Diet

Lose Up to 18 Pounds, Reverse Wrinkles,
and Improve Your Health
in Just 3 Weeks

TABLE OF CONTENTS

The reproduction, duplication or transmission of any of the included information is considered illegal whether done in print or electronically. Creating a recorded copy or a secondary copy of this work is also prohibited unless the action of doing so is first cleared through the Publisher and condoned in writing. All rights reserved.

Any information contained in the following pages is considered accurate and truthful and that any liability through inattention or by any use or misuse of the topics discussed within falls solely on the reader. There are no cases in which the Publisher of this work can be held responsible or be asked to provide reparations for any loss of monetary gain or other damages which may be caused by following the presented information in any way shape or form.

The following information is presented purely for informative purposes and is therefore considered universal. The information presented within is done so without a contract or any other type of assurance as to its quality or validity.

Any trademarks which are used are done so without consent and any use of the same does not imply consent or that permission was gained from the owner. Any trademarks or brands found within are purely used for clarification purposes and no owners are in anyway affiliated with this work.

Introduction

I want to thank and congratulate you for purchasing this book, *Bone Broth Diet: Lose up to 18 Pounds, Reverse Wrinkles, and Improve Your Health in Just 3 Weeks*. With the Standard American Diet such a prevalent issue in many first world countries, this book and others like it are the first step toward extricating yourself from a system designed to keep you hooked on processed foods, whatever the cost.

This book contains proven steps and strategies on how to use the Paleo diet and one of its key components, bone broth, to get in shape and to look and feel younger than you have in years. While a cup of bone broth a day has a myriad of benefits, as discussed in chapters 3 and 4, to truly turn your life around, you should consider the Paleo diet. While the Paleo diet does involve giving up most, if not all, refined carbohydrates, the benefits will most definitely outweigh the sacrifice. Changing your diet can be difficult, but keep at it; the results are worth it.

Thanks again for purchasing this book, I hope you enjoy it!

Chapter 1

Why the Standard American Diet Stinks

Compared to diets in many other developed countries, the diet of most American's isn't just less healthy, it is practically deadly. This diet is referred to as the Standard American Diet by nutritionists, and it includes too much saturated fat, more than a healthy amount of fats from animals, and more than a healthy amount of processed foods. At the same time, it contains a less than healthy amount of fiber, only a small amount of plants, and hardly any complex carbohydrates. As such, nutritionists have determined that the Standard American Diet leads to an increased risk of cancer, heart disease, and stroke.

Between 1970 and 2008, the Standard American Diet ballooned in size, increasing its total calorie count by more than 25 percent. Likewise, studies have shown that within that period, the number of times the average American ate at a fast food "restaurant" grew by 75 percent. Even worse, more than half of those meals included unhealthy hamburgers, and more than 30 percent included an extra sugary soda. These sodas are loaded with high fructose corn syrup, which is significantly less healthy than the complex carbohydrates Americans should be consuming instead.

Recent studies have shown that as soon as a new region develops eating habits associated with the Standard American Diet, the population's average chance of developing cancer, heart disease, and stroke double within three to five years. Meanwhile, countries who follow the opposite of the Standard American Diet, one which incorporates a lot of fiber while remaining low in fat and including a lot of plants and complex carbohydrates, retain a lower risk for all three types of illness.

It is ironic that the United States spends countless dollars on cancer research when a measurable way to reduce the risk of cancer is staring scientists in the face every day as they head out to lunch. America has become a fast food culture, failing to account for the fact that quality is as important as quantity when it comes to the carbohydrates, proteins, and fats which are churned out in fast food chains and consumed by unthinking millions every day. Nutritionists say those who replace their fat-saturated diets with a diet including leafy greens, nuts, and fish will decrease their chance of heart disease by five percent for every one percent of saturated fat that is replaced.

Another major issue with the Standard American Diet is the way in which it relies upon processed foods. Any foodstuff can be considered processed if it has been treated with chemicals in some way. A list of processed foods would also include those which are made with refined ingredients or those which are entirely artificially created. Only when all the ingredients in a foodstuff are completely free of chemicals can that item be considered truly real.

When a processed item is compared to its unprocessed counterpart, the processed version will most likely have two to three times as much sugar, either in its original form or in its no less insidious form, high fructose corn syrup. This addition serves little function, save making the item more palatable to a society addicted to sugar, while adding extra calories in the process. In a healthy and productive diet, the consumption of sugar is heavily regulated for the things it does to the metabolism. Excessive levels of sugar in your system leads directly to high levels of negative cholesterol, a buildup of fat on the liver, and, when taken to extremes, to diabetes as the body loses the ability to process insulin. In addition, studies have shown that those who eat too much sugar are at a higher risk of cancer, heart disease, and obesity.

What makes the Standard American Diet such an issue is that most of the products which it includes are formulated in such a way as to encourage the consumer to always want more and more. The reason processed foods are addictive is because of the way the primal human brain is wired. Back in the distant past, our ancestors learned that foods which were full of fats, sugars, or salts would keep them alive longer because these things tended to also have more of the nutrients the human body needs to survive. These days however, the opposite is true and foods high in fats, sugars, and salts rarely contain any health benefits whatsoever.

Modern companies are aware of our brains' hardwiring and do their best to make their foods as full of the things the body craves as possible. This is why it is possible to become addicted to food or to still feel hungry after you have just eaten an entire bag of fast food. If you consume a lot of processed food regularly, be aware that it is possible for the brain to become so addicted to the chemicals supplied by the food that it stops producing those chemicals on its own. For this reason, quitting processed food can be just as difficult as quitting cigarettes or alcohol.

When looking for foods to steer clear of there are a few useful rules of thumb to remember. If an item is high in preservatives, contains chemical colors, or contains flavorings or additives to give it texture, it should be avoided at all costs; your health may depend on it. Another extremely important warning sign of an unhealthy food is when it contains a large amount of carbohydrates in their refined form.

Carbohydrates which have been refined are significantly less nutritious than the carbohydrates in healthier items, as they provide only a third of the energy of their unrefined friends. When the body breaks down refined carbohydrates, the process leads to an increase in blood sugar which ultimately leads to a sugar crash and an intense desire for additional refined carbohydrates or some other form of sugar. And finally, you guessed it, consuming a high amount of refined carbohydrates also leads to a significantly increased chance of heart disease, stroke, and cancer. Do your body a favor and start checking labels. It could be a matter of life and death.

Chapter 2

Foods to Avoid

Despite the fact that the Standard American Diet is essentially an invitation to heart disease, cancer, and stroke at every turn, its omnipresence in the modern world makes it difficult, if not impossible, to avoid. To help counter this problem, the following chapter discusses a wide variety of foods and why avoiding them is most likely the healthiest course of action.

Red Meat

Despite its near universal presence in the Standard American Diet, red meat is the first thing you should avoid when turning your eating habits around. This is mainly due to a chemical compound known as carnitine, which can be found in all red meat and attacks the body in two distinct ways. First, it speeds up the process by which arteries clog. Then, it combines with intestinal bacteria to form a new compound which attacks the heart directly, immediately contributing to an increased risk of heart disease.

Processed Meat

As a general rule, meat of any variety is a terrific source of protein. However, meat which has been excessively processed, such as that which comes from fast food restaurants, is the exception to the rule. Before the meat from fast food restaurants even reaches your hands, the amount of preservatives it has absorbed negates any benefits it might have started with. What's more, the initial low quality of the meat translates to less protein than anything you would find in a grocery store. Finally, these meats are much higher in sodium, which causes heart disease, as well as an excess of nitrates, which can make it difficult for the body's red blood cells to process oxygen.

Most Potatoes

While it is true that starches are more beneficial to a healthy body than sugars, non-organic potatoes are often subjected to several pesticides and fungicides while they are still in the soil. After they are done soaking up chemicals through osmosis, they are then treated with even more chemicals to keep them fresh for as long as possible. The chemicals they are treated with have been shown to increase the consumer's risk for autism, asthma, difficult learning, defects at birth, both Parkinson's and Alzheimer's diseases, and more than one type of cancer.

Farm-Raised Salmon

Much like with processed meat, traditional salmon is a great source of protein, but salmon raised on a farm contain enough potential problems to be avoided whenever possible. When they are kept in large groups, salmon lose their nutritional value as their vitamin D levels drop. In addition, farm-raised salmon are routinely treated with DDTs, PCBs, bromine, and pesticides containing carcinogens. A steady influx of bromine in your diet has shown to cause an increased risk of mental illness and skin disorders, as well as a disruption in the way the thyroid functions, an increased chance of birth defects, and an increased risk of slower cognitive and neural development.

Most Milk

Despite its prominence in the food pyramid, milk which has not been certified organic is generally treated with several different growth hormones to make the cow produce as much as possible. While this is unfortunate, as it increases the amount of puss in every gallon of milk, it also adds quite a large amount of antibiotics to each gallon. This, in turn, can make it more difficult for the body to fight off infections in the future. The added hormones have also been shown to increase the risk of breast, prostate, and colon cancers.

Margarine

Almost since its creation, margarine spread has been billed as a healthy alternative to butter, but reality could not be further from the truth. When compared to butter, margarine contains much higher amounts of trans-fats, and excessive use of margarine has been linked to a higher chance of heart disease and diabetes.

Microwave Popcorn

While not particularly healthy, the biggest issue with microwave popcorn is the diactyl hiding in many artificial butter flavors. This chemical can cause damage to the lungs, which can lead to bronchitis or even cancer, and it hides under the "artificial flavorings" label, so there is no easy way to tell which brands use it. All popcorn is high in trans-fats, however, so it is easier to avoid the whole bad bunch.

Pop

While it is easy to see why traditional soda pop would be unhealthy, as it is literally comprised of liquid sugar, the diet or zero calorie versions contain their own dangers and should be avoided as well. The artificial sweeteners in these pop alternatives, including acesuifame-k, saccharin, cyclamate, aspartame, and sucralose, all increase blood pressure and still come with the ultimate "sugar" crash, weight gain, and increased risk of cancer that come with processed sugars.

White Flour

Despite its prevalence in nearly every aspect of the Standard American Diet, heavily refined white flour contains practically zero nutritional elements and should, therefore, be staunchly avoided. When consumed regularly, refined carbohydrates such as those found in white flower have been shown to increase the chance of breast cancer by over 200 percent.

Chapter 3

Bone Broth and the Paleo Diet Explained

While looking at the bones left over after a good meal, it can be difficult to see them as anything but detritus, but, in reality, the opposite is true. While they appear lifeless and devoid of nutrition, locked away inside them is a wide variety of delicious essential vitamins and nutrients your body will gladly absorb if given the opportunity. When prepared correctly, you will find that these leftover bones provide a delightful mix of anti-inflammatory and restorative properties, as well as fats and minerals the body needs to stay healthy. This is the reason animals the world over can be found gnawing on bones: they know what goodness hides inside. Luckily, you have an easier way of getting at the benefits than cracking the bones with your teeth.

Bone broth is an essential part of the Paleo diet, which focuses on eating the way our ancestors did thousands of years ago with a diet high in protein, nuts, seeds, fish, and leafy greens. This diet is ideal for those who do not enjoy counting calories, as the focus is instead on ensuring everything that enters the body is already beneficial, making the calorie count behind every individual item meaningless. In addition to always being healthy, a diet high in these items will help you lose weight while promoting muscle gain at the same time. If you stick with it, you will notice an increase in weight loss until your body adjusts to the new diet. Additionally, you will no longer be exposed to all of the chemicals in processed food, which make the signs of aging much more apparent.

The Paleo diet works because our early ancestors were hunter/gatherers and, despite discovering agriculture thousands of years ago, our bodies have yet to adapt too far away from that hunter/gatherer lifestyle. While we have as species moved on to revere grains extensively, our bodies only need a small amount of these items, and the general recommended daily dose of 6-11 servings is several magnitudes higher than it should be. As a result, all of these excess grains simply turn into sugar that the body has trouble dealing with.

In addition to turning into sugar, all of those carbohydrates contain gluten, to which a shocking percentage of humans are intolerant, according to recent studies. Consuming gluten if you have a gluten intolerance can lead to acid reflux, joint pain, reproductive issues, and more. Most grains contain a compound called lectin, which is a natural toxin plants have built up to discourage consumption. Grains themselves are trying to tell us to stop eating them, but the Standard American Diet persists.

Cutting out carbohydrates, processed foods, and sugars automatically decreases your chance for heart disease, cancer, and stroke, but then leaves you without the most common form of energy found in the Standard American Diet. However, the human body was not designed to run on so many carbohydrates, and after you spend a few days working through carbohydrate withdrawal, you will find your body is just as happy to burn excess fat for that energy as it was to burn carbohydrates.

While your body will still need some carbohydrates to function properly, you can easily find those in vegetables, such as sweet potatoes (a staple of the Paleo diet), and plenty of fruits. You can easily stock up on vegetables with little caloric impact, as vegetables such as broccoli boast 30 calories and 6 grams of carbs per serving. Meanwhile, most pastas include at least 200 calories per serving and a whopping 42 grams of carbs (enough for three days).

Much like with carbohydrates, the human body isn't as good at processing dairy as the Standard American Diet would suggest. In fact, the enzymes which process milk break down after childhood, and many adults have undiagnosed issues caused by drinking milk simply because we are not built to process it. Dairy is the one facet of the Paleo diet in which there is a little wiggle room. If you know your body and know that milk doesn't affect you, then it is fine in moderation. If you are unsure, it is best to cut it out just to be safe.

Paleo Diet Outline

- *Grass fed meat only:* Animals which are raised on a diet of grain can develop many of the same problems as people who eat too much of the same. What's more, by eating those animals you are allowing them to pass their issues on to you.
- *Fowl:* As long as they are certified organic and cage-free, fowl of all types are fair game.
- *Fish:* As long as they are not farm-raised, eat all the fish you want.
- *Eggs:* Organic eggs enriched with Omega-3 are the best for you.
- *Vegetables:* Eat as many organic vegetables as you can handle as long as they aren't fried.
- *Oils:* When you need to cook with oil, stick with coconut, avocado, or anything else natural.
- *Fruits:* Organic fruits are fine in moderation as they contain a fair amount of natural sugar.
- *Nuts:* Organic nuts are high in calories and energy, so they make a great post-workout snack.
- *Tubers:* As previously discussed, stay away from traditional potatoes but feel free to fill up on sweet potatoes and yams. They are high in calories and carbohydrates, so stick to a reasonable amount.

Nutrient Guidelines

While there are no strict numbers or eating regulations to go along with the Paleo diet, it is important to ensure you are getting the correct number of vitamins and minerals in your diet every day. With this in mind, use the following nutrient tips as a guideline when setting up a Paleo diet plan.

- **Base every meal around a protein:** Start with either pork, fish, chicken, or eggs.
- **Add a complimentary vegetable or fruit.**
- **Repeat.**

It really is that simple. If you find you are still feeling a little hungry after meals or don't think you are taking in enough calories every day, it is perfectly fine to add some healthy fats into the mix. Nuts are a great choice for this role, but so are things like avocado, almond butter, and coconut oil. Fruits are also a good choice in moderation as they can be high in natural sugar. Inversely, if you try the Paleo diet and do not seem to be losing weight, keep an eye on your nut and fruit intake, as those two together add up quick.

When following the Paleo diet, an important thing to consider is that fat should ideally make up a large percentage of your daily diet. You see, fat has developed somewhat of a negative reputation over the years which can be traced back to the oversimplification of what fat is and what it is good for. As it turns out, fats are an essential aspect of a healthy eating plan. They provide acids, which are crucial to keeping soft skin, vitamins that provide much-needed fuel, and omega-3 acids that improve heart health.

Even the US Department of Agriculture is on the right side of the war on fat. Their most recent round of dietary guidelines shows that, ideally, 30 percent of your diet should be made of fat.

In addition to not worrying about fats, it is important to not expect the Paleo diet to align with any specific schedule. You do not need to worry about eating every three hours or fasting for eight hours or only on weeknights that end in Y. Eat when you are hungry and stop before you feel excessively full. If you are hungry again in two hours, have a light snack. Don't worry about eating just because the clock says it is time to eat; if you don't feel hungry when dinner time comes around, skip it.

Mitigating Cost

While searching out high quality sources of vitamins and proteins can easily get expensive, that doesn't have to be the case. What follows are a number of tips for eating healthy on the cheap.

- *Make eating healthy and cheap a priority:* If you have an honest conversation with yourself about the importance of eating healthy and fully commit yourself to the task, making the extra effort to search out affordable healthy options is much easier.
- *Plan ahead:* If you don't take the time to plan out what you will be eating between grocery store visits, you will be much more likely to go off book and hit the closest fast food place for a value meal.
- *Start with the basics:* While many all-natural luxury foods fall on the expensive side, foods like rice, fruits,

vegetables, and basic meats aren't too far outside the cost for their processed brethren. If you take the time to cook all your own meals, the individual cost of each item drops significantly.

Diet Outline

Here's an example of what you might eat for one day for breakfast, lunch, dinner, a snack, and dessert.

Paleo Scramble

This mix of eggs, sausage, bacon, and salsa will have you eagerly greeting the morning sun in no time. This recipe requires about five minutes of preparation, fifteen minutes of cook time, and serves 2.

What's in it

- 1 cup of organic salsa or green chili
- 5 onions (diced)
- Organic bacon (3 strips)
- 5 pounds of organic sausage (crumbled)
- 4 organic eggs

Instructions

1. Set a burner to a middle heat.
2. Mix the bacon, sausage, and onions in a frying-pan and stir as needed for 10 minutes or until everything is evenly cooked.
3. Pour the whisked eggs over the contents of the pan.
4. Stir for another four minutes or until the eggs have finished cooking.
5. Add salsa or chili to taste.

Pesto Chicken Salad

This is an easy lunch recipe that will satisfy your daily levels of leafy greens, and it tastes great. Besides cooking the chicken, this meal only takes about 10 minutes to make and serves 2.

What's in it
- Several organic tomatoes (halved)
- 6 oz. of mixed greens
- .25 tsp. of salt
- .25 tsp. of pepper
- 2 tbsp. vinegar
- 2 tbsp. organic oil
- 3 tbsp. organic onion (chopped)
- .25 cups of pesto
- 1 chicken breast (chopped)

Instructions
- Combine the chicken, pesto, and onion in a bowl and make sure the chicken is completely covered in pesto.
- Combine the remaining items and toss the greens to ensure that they are covered completely.
- Mix all of the items together and serve.

Sweet Potato Casserole
Despite seeming rather indulgent, this casserole is filled with only the healthiest of ingredients. This recipe will be ready in just 40 minutes after only five minutes of preparation. This recipe serves 10.

What's in it

- 2 tbsp. applesauce (organic)
- 2 tbsp. maple syrup (organic)
- 2 tbsp. coconut flour
- 2 tbsp. coconut sugar
- 3 tbsp. pepitas
- 1 tsp. of vanilla
- .5 cups of coconut cream
- 2 chopped sweet potatoes

Instructions

1. Boil potatoes.
2. Heat the oven to 350 degrees.
3. Mix the potatoes with the vanilla, salt, and coconut cream.
4. Put the result in a casserole dish and bake for 24 minutes or until brown.
5. When the casserole is finished, spread the remaining items on top and serve.

Chips

These Paleo chips make a great healthy snack in moderation.

What's in it

- 1 tsp. of Kosher salt
- 2 tbsp. of coconut oil
- .5 cups of water
- 1 tsp. of onion (powdered)
- 1 tsp. of garlic (powdered)

- 1 tsp. of organic green chili (powdered)
- .5 cups of sunflower seeds
- .5 cups of sesame seeds
- .5 cups of flax seeds
- .5 cups of almond flour

Instructions
- Heat the oven to 375 degrees.
- Line a baking sheet with parchment.
- Combine the dry ingredients.
- Add water and oil with the other dry ingredients.
- Place a single tbsp.'s amount of the mixture across the baking sheet.
- Cover with parchment.
- The chips should be ready after 15 minutes in the oven.

Cherry Pie Bars

Just because you have found a new and healthy way to eat doesn't mean you can't have a dessert now and then. When eaten in moderation, there is nothing wrong with a healthy dessert at the end of a long day. This recipe will be ready to go in just 10 minutes, and the recipe makes roughly 20 squares.

What's in it
- 1.5 cups of cherries (dried)
- 1.4 cups of almonds (raw)
- 10 dates (no pits)

Instructions

- Combine all three ingredients using a food processor.
- Add water until the mix starts to clump together.
- Place the clumps into a lined baking dish and place the dish in the refrigerator until it is firm.

Why It Works

Remember, the whole of the Paleo diet is in sticking to a set group of foods; you don't need to worry about eating too much (within moderation), or about scheduling cheat days, or counting calories, or dealing with complicated point systems. The diet is effective because the types of food it contains are guaranteed to be both nutritious and filling, which makes it difficult for most people to overeat.

Picture it this way: if you wanted to consume the caloric equivalent of a "snack" sized bag of chips, you would have to eat close to two dozen stalks of broccoli. Now ask yourself how much broccoli you could eat before feeling full. That, in a nutshell (pun intended), is what makes the Paleo diet so effective; it self-corrects negative habits. Even better, once you start, you never feel hungry. A plate of vegetables and a small portion of meat will leave you feeling full for several times as long as something full of processed chemicals.

If you feel as though the thought of giving up all those delicious carbohydrates and processed foods is too much too bear, then the Paleo diet might not be for you. It is as simple as that. However, before you give it up entirely, ask yourself a few questions first. Do you struggle with weight loss? Do you feel as though you have enough energy throughout the day? How many cups of coffee do you drink a day? How do you feel about counting calories?

Depending on how you answered these questions, there is a very real chance that the Paleo diet may be just the thing you are looking for. Do yourself a favor and try it for just one month. A month is enough time for your body to stop freaking out over the radical change in diet you have experienced and start operating on the fuel the human body has known since we learned to hunt and gather. After 30 days, take stock of how you feel and then make a well-informed decision from there.

If you are interested in seeing how your body reacts to the Paleo diet but just can't give up the carbohydrates, then take it slow. Dieting doesn't have to be a scenario in which a single failure results in a complete loss; it is about changing the way you think about food and creating new, healthy routines. If carbohydrates are a deal breaker for you, then start cutting them back slowly instead of all at once. Don't feel guilty about the substitution either, as that guilt will make it easier to slip back into old habits. If you start to feel guilty about eating a few carbohydrates, just remind yourself how much better you are eating now compared to how you were eating before. Take it one day at a time. Dieting is not a race.

Chapter 4

Best Bone Broth Recipes

Bone broth is an essential element of the Paleo diet because of the myriad of health benefits and nutritional staples it contains. Bone broth has always been a staple of non-Standard American Diets the world over. The health benefits found in bone broth are substantial, and the following are just a few of the reasons it is considered a core part of the Paleo diet.

- **Get your gut into shape:** A 2014 study on bone broth found that as little as a single cut of bone broth per day is enough to counteract any symptoms of leaky gut syndrome, because the gelatin in the bones naturally seals any holes in the intestines. It is also good for coating the intestines to prevent leaky gut syndrome. In addition, it helps with issues of chronic diarrhea, food intolerance, and chronic constipation.

- **Keep your joints healthy:** Bone broth contains a lot of glucosamine and gelatin, both of which have been proven to reduce joint pain and to maintain healthy joints. What's more, a compound in bone broth called chondroitin sulfate has been shown to help prevent osteoarthritis.

- **Look younger:** Bone broth has been shown to be an ample source of collagen, which is known to aid skin in looking younger and more radiant. Getting an extra supply of collagen from bone broth is significantly cheaper than having it injected manually. In addition, collagen helps make your nails harder and your hair shiny and more radiant.

- **Improve your sleep:** Bone broth contains glycine, which studies have shown aids in providing a solid, restful night's sleep. As an added bonus, it has been shown to improve memory and increase focus.

- **Beef up your immune system:** Bone broth is often considered a super-food thanks to the wide variety of healthy minerals that can be found within it. As common sense has always held, chicken soup is good for increasing the immune system.

- **Strengthen your bones:** Bone broth contains high amounts of calcium, magnesium, and phosphorous, which are all things your own bones need.

- **Increase your energy:** Drinking bone broth has been empirically shown to provide an almost immediate energy boost, though the science behind why this happens is still being determined. Try it for yourself, however, and you won't be able to deny how much more energized you feel.

Bones are high in protein, roughly 50 percent by volume. Collagen, which provides the protein matrix in the bones, becomes gelatin when cooked and is the reason cooked broth hardens in the fridge. Gelatin contains two important amino acids, proline and glycine, which perform several critical functions when ingested. Perhaps most importantly, they provide the body with the base elements to repair damaged connective tissue, including the tendons in charge of connecting muscle and bone. If you are interested in increasing how much you can lift at the gym, add a cup of bone broth to your pre-gym workout.

In addition to aiding in the repair of damaged ligaments, proteins found in bone broth provide an astounding benefit to those suffering from rheumatoid arthritis and other chronic autoimmune diseases. When it comes to arthritis, these proteins can help mitigate the response from the body which causes the disease and even, in some cases, reverse the symptoms significantly. A recent study found that when given a regular supplement of chicken collagen, 60 out of 60 patients saw an improvement, and four patients even went into complete remission.

Another reason bone broth is so beneficial for maintaining healthy joints is thanks to the high amount of glycosaminoglycans (GAGs) found in the broth. GAGs are extremely beneficial carbohydrates common in connective tissue and bones and has been shown to reduce the symptoms of painful joints. One particular GAG, hyaluronic acid, has been shown to help prevent osteoarthritis even when not directly injected into the affected area. Finally, the GAG chondroitin sulfate has shown promising results when it is used to repair and reduce the damage done by arthritis.

The most famous GAG is called glucosamine, which is a common vitamin supplement aimed at improving joint health and decreasing pain. There is as much glucosamine in a cup of bone broth as in any daily supplement. If you routinely find yourself in situations in which you and your joints take a beating, starting to drink a cup of bone broth a day might be one of the healthiest things you can do.

In addition to its benefits to joint health, the best part about bone broth is the benefits it brings to even the healthiest digestive tract. In addition to helping you sleep, glycine helps ensure a regular flow of stomach acid. What's more, glycine is a key part of bile which is used to digest fat in the small intestine and improve cholesterol levels.

A lesser known aspect of the anti-inflammatory property of bone broth is that the proteins found in the broth have been shown to help athletes recover faster after a serious injury. This is due to the fact that in times of stress or injury, the body has a natural need for more amino acids than normal. This need is easily filled by bone broth as it is full of several nutrients that aren't considered essential because the body creates them naturally, but they are still nice to have around during an emergency.

The biggest contributors in these situations are glutamine and arginine. In addition to supporting bone and tissue regeneration, these amino acids help wounds to heal faster and to leave less scarring by increasing the production of collagen. This is done by converting proline, another compound found in the body, through a process that is not yet completely understood.

Another lesser known benefit of bone broth is the fact that glycine acts as a neurotransmitter inhibitor. This means it helps you relax while easing your aches and pains.

Bone broth's myriad of restorative benefits also extend to improving the detoxification process, because glycine aids the liver in removing especially harmful toxins. It can also help dissolve the fatty deposits added to the liver by a strict adherence to the Standard American Diet. Glycine pulls double duty again by being a required component for the synthesis of glutathione, a uric acid crucial to allowing the body to create its own antioxidants. Increasing the amount of glutathione essentially boosts levels of Vitamin C, which in turn cuts down on oxidative based stressors. Finally, maintaining a high level of glycine keeps the body's levels of methionine in check, which is key to maintaining a blood level balance and keeping the body's levels of B vitamins in check.

All of these benefits are seen before the marrow itself is taken into account. Bone marrow is a key component of the immune system and also contains a variety of cells which strengthen bones and boost immune functions. In addition to marrow, the bones themselves offer a wide variety of minerals based on the type of animal they previously belonged to. Bones from cows and pigs are high in potassium, magnesium, and calcium, fish bones are high in iodine, and the bones of fowl contain extra potassium and calcium.

Because every bone is different, it can be difficult to say how much of what minerals make it into any one batch of broth. The quality of life the animal led prior to its death goes a long way toward determining the nutritional content of its bones. With that being said, there are a few simple ways to ensure that your broth is as high in mineral content as possible. The easiest option is to always remember to include at least a tablespoon of an acidic element to your broth to help dissolve the bones. Another easy solution is to simply eat the smaller bones along with the broth. While this may seem odd, after cooking for so long, the smaller bones will be crunchy and dissolve easily on the tongue. Another option, if you do not like the texture of the bones, is to simply grind them up as soon as they are done cooking and add the powder back into the broth before you cool it.

Bone Broth Recipes

Finding the bones for your broth might just be the hardest part of the entire endeavor. To start, try the butcher section of your local grocery store or an Asian food market. The tougher the bone, the better. Chicken's feet, oxtails, chicken necks, beef knuckles, and, of course, soup bones will all do the trick nicely. As stands to reason, the bones from grass-fed animals are preferable to other varieties, though it can be difficult to source your bones. When looking for grass-fed bones, the companies Tropical Traditions and U.S. Wellness Meats are good places to start.

To keep your broth tasting great for as long as possible, it is important to cool all of your broth as soon as it has been cooked before placing it in an airtight container (or two). Keep a three-day supply in the refrigerator and keep the rest in the freezer. Remember to always heat the broth before eating as cold broth congeals from all the healthy nutrients inside.

Basic Bone Broth

This basic bone broth can serve as a template from which to build other broths. The recipe makes three to four servings.

What's in it

- 2 lbs. of bones
- 1 tbsp. of apple cider vinegar
- Vegetables to taste

Instructions

1. Place the bones in a crockpot full of cold water. Bones can be roasted to create a heartier broth.

2. Add the apple cider vinegar. This step is crucial as the vinegar aids in pulling as much nutrients as possible from the bone.
3. Add vegetables to taste. Herbs, pepper, onions, and a clove of garlic are a nice start.
4. Set the crockpot to simmer. Four hours are required for chicken and fish bone broth, while beef bones require a minimum of six hours. Between 24 and 48 hours is considered the appropriate amount of time required to pull all the nutrients from the bones.

Beef Bone Broth

Before you begin preparing this filling bone broth, roast the bones with your favorite vegetables to give the broth an extra boost. This recipe makes about 8 cups of broth.

What's in it

- 1 tbsp. of apple cider vinegar
- 2 tbsp. of black pepper
- 2 bay leaves
- 2 celery stalks (2-inch pieces)
- 1 clove of garlic (halved)
- 1 onion (quartered)
- 1 leek (2-inch pieces)
- 2 carrots (2-inch pieces)
- 4 lbs. of beef bones (a mix of oxtail, knuckle, short rib, and marrow bones is preferred)

Instructions

1. Ensure that your oven has been preheated to 450 degrees Fahrenheit before placing the bones, leek, onion, carrots, and garlic on a baking sheet. Bake for 20 minutes.
2. Toss the items on the pan and roast for another 15 minutes or until the contents are a roasted brown.
3. Fill your crockpot with cool water before adding the vinegar, peppercorn, bay leaves, and celery. Add the roasted items. Ensure you have enough water to cover all the vegetables and bones.
4. Bring the pot to a boil after replacing the lid. Once the contents have boiled, reduce the heat to a low setting and cook for 24 to 48 hours.

Chicken Bone Broth

After just one sip of this chicken bone broth, you will swear off store-bought chicken soup for ever. This recipe makes about eight cups of broth.

What's in it

- 3 chicken carcasses (roasted)
- 1 tbsp. of apple cider vinegar
- 1 bay leaf (chopped)
- 2 onions (halved)
- 1 clove of garlic
- 2 tbsp. of peppercorns (ground)
- 3 celery stalks (chopped)
- 3 carrots (chopped)
- Parsley (to taste)

- Thyme (to taste)

Instructions

1. Assemble all of the ingredients and place them in the crockpot (a 6-quart crockpot will hold all of the items plus the 2.5 quarts of water required).
2. Set the crockpot on a low setting and cook for 24 to 48 hours.
3. If you are interested in straining out the excess fat, pour the contents through a wire strainer before cooling and storing.
4. Note on storing: if your broth doesn't gel as discussed, it is most likely because you added too much water. Cut back next time to increase the nutritional value per cup.

Turkey Bone Broth

This bone broth is a great answer to what to do with holiday leftovers. This recipe makes about eight cups of broth.

What's in it

- 1 large turkey carcass
- 1 tbsp. of apple cider vinegar
- 2 tbsp. of black pepper
- 2 bay leaves
- 2 celery stalks (2-inch pieces)
- 1 clove of garlic (halved)
- 1 onion (quartered)
- 1 leek (2-inch pieces)

- 2 carrots (2-inch pieces)

Instructions

1. Assemble all of the ingredients and place them in the crockpot (a 6-quart crockpot will hold all of the items plus the 2.5 quarts of water required).
2. Set the crockpot on a low setting and cook for 24 to 48 hours.
3. If you are interested in straining out the excess fat, pour the contents through a wire strainer before cooling and storing.

Fish Bone Broth

There is some debate as to which fish bones make the best broth, though white fish is generally preferred. What is important to remember is to include all the heads and fins, but removing the eyes is optional. This recipe makes about 8 cups.

What's in it

- 2 lbs. of fish remains
- .25 cups of apple cider vinegar
- Sea salt to taste

Instructions

1. Place 3 quarts of water along with the fish bits in a stockpot that holds at least 4 quarts.
2. Add the vinegar before bringing the water to a boil.

3. While the items are boiling, foam will rise to the top of the water. Always remove this foam as it is the impurities in the fish leaving the broth.
4. Reduce the heat and let the pot simmer for up to 24 hours.

Pork Bone Broth

Pork bones often offer a cheaper alternative to beef bone and cost around half as much on average. Pork stock tends to be fattier than other stocks and should be strained before and after it has been in the refrigerator. This recipe makes about two quarts of broth.

What's in it

- 3 lbs. of pork bones
- 1 tbsp. of apple cider vinegar
- Peppercorns (ground)
- Pinch of sea salt

Instructions

1. Assemble all of the ingredients and place them in the crockpot (a 6-quart crockpot will hold all of the items plus the 2.5 quarts of water required).
2. Set the crockpot on a low setting and cook for 24 to 48 hours.

Conclusion

Thank you again for purchasing this book! I hope it was able to inform you on the myriad of benefits that come from eating a cup of bone broth per day and of the Paleo diet at large. Transitioning away from the Standard American Diet can be difficult, but once you are free you will soon begin to see and feel a wide variety of benefits. You will look and feel healthier and younger than you have in years.

The next step is to stop reading already and to get out into the real world and start eating healthier. There will always be excuses as to why you "can't" eat healthy, but you should ignore them and start tomorrow. A happier, healthier you will thank you.

Finally, if you enjoyed this book, I'd like to ask you for a favor. Would you be kind enough to leave a review for this book on Amazon? It would be greatly appreciated!

Thank you again for purchasing this book!

I hope this book helped you to understand how bone broth will benefit you.

The next step is to implement what you have learned.

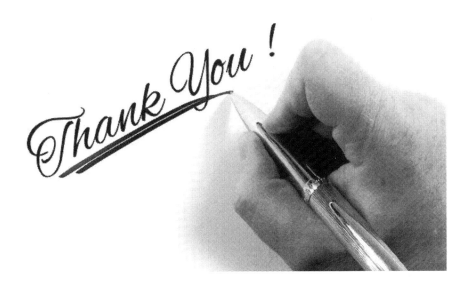

Finally, if you enjoyed this book, would you be kind enough to leave a review for this book on Amazon?

Thank you and good luck!

Made in the USA
Monee, IL
24 June 2022